al yourself
with

reflexology

Chris Stormer

Hodder Education
338 Euston Road, London NW1 3BH.

Hodder Education is an Hachette UK company

First published in UK 2011 by Hodder Education.

This edition published 2011.

Copyright © Chris Stormer

www.hoddereducation.co.uk

Typeset by MPS Limited, a Macmillan Company.
Printed in Great Britain by CPI Cox & Wyman, Reading.

Contents

reflexology at a glance

When humans first set foot on earth, their feet were naturally stimulated by the ground's undulating surfaces, giving their inner being time to adjust to life's 'ups and downs'. However, with footwear forming an unnatural and inhibitive barrier between the soles and the inner essence, it's hardly surprising that there are so many 'lost' souls wandering aimlessly around trying to 'find their feet'.

In a vain and desperate attempt to fit in, many people impose deplorable demands on themselves, as well as others, and succumb to the constant pressure of trying to be the person that society wants them to be by conforming to unrealistic conditioned belief systems that don't necessarily suit them. Can you imagine the impact and adverse implications that this must have, not just on the body, but also on the feet? Fortunately there is a solution! Reflexology balances the whole for greater progress every step of the way.

Reflexology is a natural form of healing that is non-invasive, simple and safe to give, yet it is responsible for some of the most impressive reactions. It does this by alerting latent healing abilities within the body through the firm but gentle massage of the feet, creating greater peace and harmony within – the most ideal environment for healing and health. As the reflexes on the feet are massaged, the corresponding parts of the body are either aroused or pacified, while, at the same time, tension is eased in the physical body, mental chatter is stilled and fraught emotions soothed.

The relaxation aspect of reflexology is important since it is only when truly relaxed and at ease that mind, body and soul can determine how best to regain and retain excellent health. At times of not feeling so good, reflexology has much to offer since it relieves discomfort from aches, pains or cramps. Its effectiveness comes from getting to the very root of the issue, so that the distressing memory associated with the symptom can be sorted out and eliminated once and for all. The beneficial effects continue from there. Fatigue, tiredness and exhaustion are counteracted; nervousness, concern, worry or fear are soothed and undue distress alleviated. In the process the whole body is cleared of impure thoughts and toxic emotions, circulation improves, underactive or sluggish areas are stimulated and hyperactive or over-productive parts are calmed. This prevents any further drain of energy, allowing equilibrium to be re-established.

Ongoing benefits

Once feeling better, reflexology is one of the best ways to stay in tip-top condition, but regular top-ups are required – ideally once a week – to keep it that way. A one-off session is great for getting back on track but it's staying there that makes all the difference. By rejuvenating and re-energizing all the cells, it increases vitality, boosts confidence and ensures a good night's sleep. It also re-establishes inner and outer trust, making it then possible to focus on what's important in life. With such an incredible sense of wellbeing, and feeling so complete, a more fulfilling and rewarding lifestyle is possible. Reflexology provides the courage and wisdom to cope with any perceived adversity and the opportunity to be authentic for ongoing transformation, growth and progress.

Advantages of learning reflexology

There are many advantages to learning and giving reflexology, especially since anybody can do it, if they so wish. It can also be given anywhere, at any time, because all that's needed are your hands and the recipient's feet. Furthermore, since only the feet are exposed, there is no embarrassment, self-consciousness or fear of feeling vulnerable. Painful body parts remain undisturbed, yet still benefit from the relief of having their related reflexes massaged. The massage itself generally takes around an hour, yet its effects last much longer.

Build-up of detrimental feelings

Whenever detrimental feelings build up inside, they invariably get in the way, causing excessive anxiety and unbearable tension. The more these noxious notions are contained, the more discernible they become, hampering progress every step of the way, no matter what. The physical tension is often too much for the body, especially when its scope of movement and ability to function become increasingly limited. Things can get so bad that there's a tendency to overreact to everything. Feeling hopeless and helpless just makes matters worse, and can even lead to the abuse of substances.

Health – the natural state of the body

The good news is that no matter how bad things have become, the body will do whatever it can to be healthy. Reflexology is always more than happy to give a helping hand.

Whatever disturbs the mind also upsets the body, causing varying degrees of discomfort. This determines the type of symptom experienced, which then invariably shows up on the feet. The point is that illness does not just randomly pick any part of the body in which to create havoc; it is, in fact, the other way round. Chaos in the mind disturbs the related part or parts of the body and is reflected onto the relevant areas of the feet, especially when the issue becomes problematic. It's the body's way of showing that something has to be done to make things better.

Whenever there's a crisis, reflexology knows how to deal with the uneasiness that comes from disturbing memories and assists in coming to terms with the traumas of the past, regardless of how devastating they may have been. For total relief from any form of discomfort, there has to be a complete shift of mindset and a favourable change of attitude.

Reflexology is a great preventative too can pick up and sort out disturbances in the mind, long before the body becomes upset. It does this by directing vital life forces through energy pathways, immediately dissipating energetic hindrances and flushing out mental and emotional congestion. With less pressure on the mind, the body can relax and function so much better, as the surge of new-found energy infiltrates the whole being. Having said this though, when first giving or receiving reflexology, there may be a feeling of exhaustion and lethargy as old, stale energies that have been suppressed for some time, begin to surface. However, once the body's natural healing resources 'kick in', the feeling of wellbeing is so tremendous that no form of adversity, no matter how serious, gets in the way for too long.

Who benefits from reflexology?

Anybody and everybody can enjoy and derive enormous benefits from reflexology, since it enables each individual to find their own inner peace. Reflexology is a non-invasive therapy that should be applied sensitively and gently to avoid unnecessary discomfort.

Be wary, though, of massaging the feet when there's a deep vein thrombosis because, as the muscles relax, the blood clot, usually in the legs, could become dislodged and travel to the lungs or heart, with the remote possibility of a stroke, pulmonary embolism or heart attack. Although there is no report of such an occurrence, it is still advisable to be cautious.

Reflexology is particularly beneficial when stuck in a rut, lacking direction, feeling alone or misunderstood or when constantly questioning, 'What on earth is the world coming to?'

A closer look at reflexology

The extraordinary and often miraculous ways in which reflexology rejuvenates, refreshes and restores cannot be fully explained, since, like any form of healing, it ultimately comes from the universe. To get an idea of what happens, think of the impact distress has on the mind, body and soul. Fear, anxiety and distrust can have such a devastating effect on the insides, physically, mentally, emotionally and spiritually, that the body instinctively defends itself. With further uneasiness and tension, the likelihood of adverse reactions increases with the muscles contracting and clamping mercilessly down on the internal organs and glands. The reduced mobility holds everything back, depriving the cells of their full quota of blood, starving them of their vital life force energies. Feeling more and more overwhelmed and overly burdened can make the feet swell and possibly harden to cover up or conceal any vulnerability. This is a good time to help the body out through the feet.

Massaging the feet entices the recipient into drifting off into the most exquisite and deeply relaxing alpha state of consciousness – the tranquility enjoyed between wakefulness and sleep. The body is then able to completely rejuvenate itself through the ongoing formation of billions of new cells that keep everything in excellent working condition.

Body reflections

Reflexology is based on the principle that the whole physical body is mapped out on a much smaller scale, over both of the feet. Everything, from the liver to the eyes to the elbows, has a specific reflex point or area on the foot linking it directly to the corresponding part or area of the body. Massaging these reflexes brings about an appropriate reaction in the body and this is when healing begins.

But having its origins in knowledge that has been handed down, from generation to generation, for thousands of years, it's inevitable that the interpretation of the reflexes varies, according to each individual's understanding.

Also, many of the organs, glands and parts overlap in the body, which means that there can be a host of reflexes in a specific part of the foot. Furthermore, there is more than one way to access a reflex, either directly via the primary reflex, or indirectly through its secondary or indirect reflex, in line with the direct reflex, on the opposite side of the foot. The two feet together represent the whole body, with the front mirrored onto the soles and the back depicted on top. The right side of the body is reflected onto the right foot, while the left foot corresponds with the left side of the body.

The face is represented on the cushioned toe pads, with each toe revealing a different aspect of the multi-dimensional mind. Moving down the feet, the toe necks mirror the neck and throat, while the balls of the feet reflect the breasts and chest. The abdominal cavity is portrayed in the fleshy parts of the insteps, whereas the denseness of the heels resembles the firmness of the bony pelvis.

The upper surfaces of the feet are solid and firm, just like the back of the body, which they so accurately reflect.

The power of your touch

Your personal touch is the most important aspect of reflexology since your touch is unique. The recipient picks up on your feelings the moment you touch them; therefore always be conscious of where you are emotionally. Take in some deep breaths and centre yourself, before massaging the feet.

When giving reflexology, touch others with supreme sensitivity, the purest of intent and complete acceptance of who and what they are.

As you touch the recipient's feet, you'll soon know how to tune into their energies and innately know how to touch them, whether it should be firm, medium or light. The desire to be touched and nurtured increases during times of illness, distress or insecurity, which is why the therapeutic touch is particularly beneficial.

When giving reflexology, use all your fingers, as well as both thumbs, because each digit has its own unique energy. This alters the vibration as well as the effect of your touch. It also introduces a far greater range of healing possibilities, enhancing the overall effect of the massage. Your thumbs help in re-establishing trust. Your index fingers encourage the recipient to get in touch with their innermost feelings. Your middle fingers activate their mind so that they know exactly what to do. Your ring fingers urge them to relate to new concepts. As for your powerful little fingers, they encourage the recipient to expand beyond tried and tested boundaries to become more of themselves. All in all, your digits make an amazing team for bringing out the very best in others.

Whether reflexology is given to ease specific symptoms or to maintain health, for the best possible results, massage every single reflex thoroughly, with a combination of all four movements (Chapter 2). Also spend extra time on congested, swollen areas or parts that lack energy and vibrancy, which are easy enough to feel. On all these areas, lightly rest a digit and gently, but firmly, 'pump' the reflex until a gush of energy is felt. Even if you can't feel anything, don't worry; the body knows exactly what to do, thanks to the impetus that you give it through touching the feet.

Within minutes there can be such great shifts in energy that, by the end of one session, the benefits are already obvious. Not taking credit for the healing means that you won't lose confidence when, from time to time, the recipient chooses not to recover from life's events.

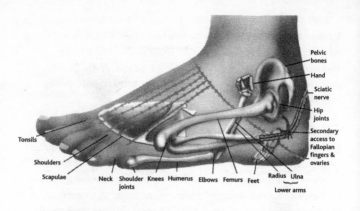

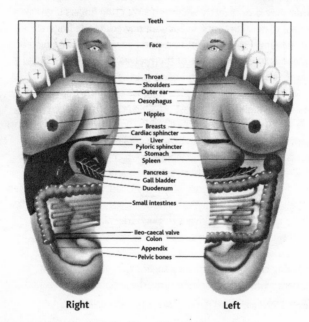

Right   **Left**

Figure 1.1 *The reflection of bodily parts in miniature on the feet.*

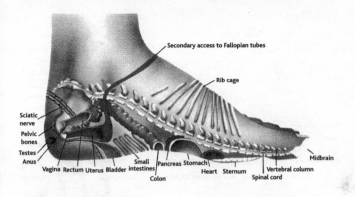

Secondary access to Fallopian tubes

Rib cage

Sciatic nerve

Pelvic bones

Testes

Anus

Vagina Rectum Uterus Bladder

Small intestines

Colon

Pancreas Stomach

Heart Sternum

Spinal cord

Vertebral column

Midbrain

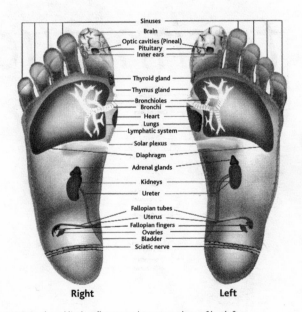

Sinuses
Brain
Optic cavities (Pineal)
Pituitary
Inner ears
Thyroid gland
Thymus gland
Bronchioles
Bronchi
Heart
Lungs
Lymphatic system
Solar plexus
Diaphragm
Adrenal glands
Kidneys
Ureter
Fallopian tubes
Uterus
Fallopian fingers
Ovaries
Bladder
Sciatic nerve

Right   **Left**

Figure 1.2 *Rack and limb reflexes on the outer edges of both feet.*

2

the technique

There is a similarity between the reflexology technique and the simple action of turning on a light! Just as a finger is placed onto the light switch in one part of a room, so it is in reflexology that a digit is placed onto a reflex on the foot. Then, just as a flick of the switch causes a light to go on elsewhere, so a slight movement of the digit on the foot initiates a reaction in the related part of the body. Even though light emanates from a small bulb, its illumination spreads far and wide. In the same way the effect of touching a reflex on the feet not only has a powerful influence on the related organ or gland, but permeates body, mind and spirit, clearing the way for new refreshing energy. Furthermore, just as the light continues to shine once the finger is taken off the switch, so too does the energy remain in the body after the digit is taken off the foot.

There are four simple movements, each of which can be adjusted to meet the ever-changing needs of the recipient. Knowing exactly how much pressure to apply is an intuitive process that cannot be taught; you will just know when to be firm, or when to pull back until there's little or no physical contact. To get a feel for these movements, try practising them on your hand first to gain the confidence to do it on others.

Technique 1 – rotation

Gently rest the tip of any digit onto the reflex (Figure 2.1) and apply slight pressure; hold for a while, then very slowly release. Without moving your digit, gently gyrate it and keep doing this for as long as necessary. Now allow your digit to rest very lightly on the skin's surface for a short while before moving it on to the next reflex. It's an ideal technique for opening up and activating all energy channels, soothing fraught nerves, creating greater awareness of oneself and others while balancing and harmonizing the whole being.

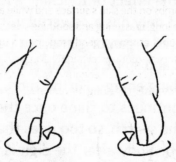

Figure 2.1 *The rotation technique.*

Technique 2 – caterpillar movement

Place the tip of your thumb gently onto the reflex and then slowly lower your thumb onto its pad (Figure 2.2) 'jerking it' fractionally forward; now raise your thumb up onto its tip again before 'dropping' it back down onto its pad. Keep rocking your thumb, up and down, as you gradually move it, bit by bit, either backwards, to unravel the past, or forwards, to ensure that progress is made. 'Walking' the thumbs eases muscular tension, relieves physical distress and alleviates aches and pains.

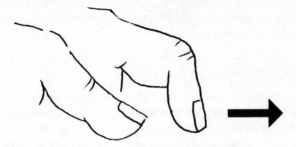

Figure 2.2 *The caterpillar movement.*

Technique 3 – stroking or milking

This technique follows the rotation and caterpillar movements. Place both thumbs on the skin's surface and while applying slight pressure, make long, reassuring and soothing sweeps (Figure 2.3), thumb over thumb, as though gently squeezing a tube of toothpaste to soothe disturbed emotions, eliminate disruptive feelings, boost self-confidence and create inner harmony. Alternatively do this technique with shorter caressing movements (Figure 2.4).

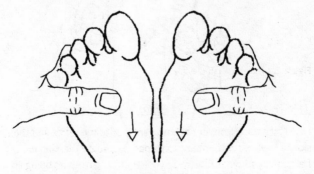

Figure 2.3 *The stroking or milking method 1.*

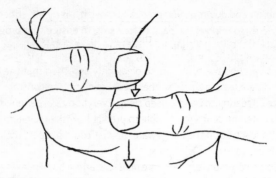

Figure 2.4 *The stroking or milking method 2.*

Technique 4 – feathering or healing caress

This is the final movement of each sequence. Very lightly stroke the skin's surface, by alternating your digits (Figure 2.5), either in generous scoops or minuscule strokes, as though you are caressing the energies just above the skin's surface to help the recipient get to know themselves and others better.

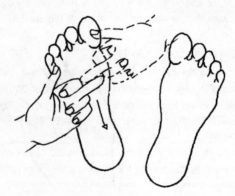

Figure 2.5 *The feathering or healing caress.*

What to expect

As the recipient drifts into the exquisite alpha level of consciousness, they remain acutely aware of everything that is going on around them, but are so pleasantly detached that they couldn't care less! In this way, they never need to lose control, despite appearing to be in a deep sleep. Everybody's experience is totally different, so it's impossible to predict how the recipient is going to react; but if they are aware of what could happen, their mind is put to rest.

Some common responses are *heat loss*, as the body relaxes and 'let's off steam'; *extreme tenderness*, despite the light touch, as hurt feelings surface; a *sinking feeling*, as mind and body drop off into a space of peace; a *floating sensation*, as burdens dissipate and a weight is taken off their whole being; *twitching* and *jerking* as a sudden surge of energy reaches previously deprived, tense areas; *pins and needles* or *numbness* in the hands coming from letting go of the difficulty in handling certain circumstances; *snoring* as deeply suppressed emotions finally escape; *visions of colours*, ranging from subdued, subtle hues to gorgeous bright tints, even though the eyes are closed.

While the feet are being massaged, the breathing can become so shallow that, at times, it is almost indiscernible, but don't panic! The recipient drifts into other spheres of consciousness, which is why it is necessary to ask them to take three deep breaths, at the end of the session, to bring them back.

Pleasurable after-effects

Most people feel absolutely fantastic after a session; full of energy along with a huge sense of relief! The renewed enthusiasm for life makes it easier to think more clearly, encourages greater tolerance and helps them to sleep much better so that they wake up feeling refreshed.

Massaging the feet effectively evacuates old, outdated beliefs and detrimental habits, making the way clear for a fresh start, which although initially disturbing, exhausting or disruptive, leaves a fantastic feeling of liberation and release.

Unusual reactions

It is impossible to cause any harm with the light, but firm, movements used in reflexology. However, individuals do like to challenge themselves, from time to time, so if this happens just remain calm and immediately place your thumbs or middle fingers onto the solar plexus reflexes (Chapter 4), and trust that you'll be intuitively guided into knowing what to do next. Encourage the recipient to drink more purified water than usual, to flush out all the additional toxins. Also suggest a further treatment, within the next day or two, to balance mind, body and soul. Although this is not a common occurrence, it is best to be aware of what to do, should there ever be an unusual and intense reaction.

Preparing for the reflexology massage

Fortunately, you have all that's needed when it comes to doing reflexology; your hands and your heart are the two most essential requirements.

A peaceful setting, in a subdued environment, allows the recipient to escape the frenetic hustle and bustle of the outside world and totally relax. Once they visually let go, by shutting their eyes, its easier for reflexology to step in and induce inner harmony.

Before beginning, give the recipient a simple and clear explanation to reassure and relax them.

Those on prescribed medication should advise their specialist of their intention to have reflexology so that appropriate adjustments can be made to the dosage.

Soak the recipient's feet, making sure that the water is pleasantly warm in winter and refreshingly cool in summer. Once they have dried their feet, invite them to lie as flat as possible on the bed or couch.

Place one pillow beneath their head and another one or two pillows under their knees and lower legs, so that their spine is straight and flat.

Shake powder into your hand, rub your palms together and spread it gently over both feet, going in between their toes. You are now ready to begin with the warm-up technique (Chapter 3).

Whether giving reflexology to maintain good health or to help somebody feel better about themselves, always do a complete foot massage, from top to bottom. Pay particular attention to the nervous system and solar plexus reflexes, as well as the endocrine gland and sensory reflexes, while also concentrating on any distressed reflexes.

When first making contact with the recipient, be conscious of how you feel because it sets the tone for the whole session.

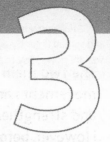

reflexology step by step

The two main effects of the reflexology movements are to either activate, tone and strengthen or pacify, calm and soothe. However, before commencing a treatment, get out of your head and into your heart. The less you consciously try, the better the treatment will be. Also avoid imposing your will. Allow yourself to be a channel for the Divine source of healing. The firm, but gentle, movements of reflexology will effectively loosen the recipient's fixation with time, encouraging them to break free from the unrealistic expectations of others. This will assist them in reconnecting, via their soles, with their true self, which means that they can then accept themselves for who and what they are. In turn, they can become more tolerant of the annoying peculiarities and actions of others. The best reactions to reflexology come from the heart, from the energy of pure love that has no expectations.

The warm-up

Start the reflexology session by using the caressing movements of the warm-up to encourage the recipient to relax. Feel free to adapt any of the following movements to make the recipient feel safe enough to let go and loosen up.

Step 1 – create trust

Take time to establish a bond so that they feel less vulnerable about baring their soles and their soul to you by gently taking the recipient's heels and resting them lightly in the palms of your hands, with their feet either covered or uncovered (Figure 3.1). As you do this, invite them to close their eyes and take in three long, deep breaths and then breathe naturally.

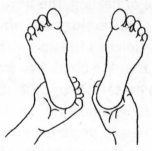

Figure 3.1 *Rest their feet in your hands.*

Step 2 – breathe and relax

As you encourage them to hold each breath for as long as possible, be aware of your own breathing and consciously relax any tension in your own body, generally in the neck, shoulders, back and upper arms.

Step 3 – caress the tops

Gently lower the recipient's heels onto the bed, then lightly but reassuringly stroke the tops of their feet, hand over hand, towards yourself (Figure 3.2), first on their right foot, then on their left to give the recipient time to get used to your energy.

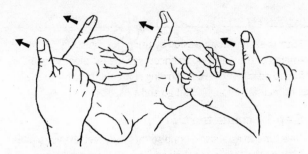

Figure 3.2 *Caress the tops.*

Step 4 – stroke their soles

Next stroke the soles of their right foot, and then of their left foot, with the backs of your hands (Figure 3.3), this time towards the recipient.

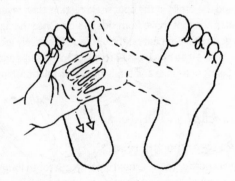

Figure 3.3 *Stroke the soles.*

Step 5 – circle the ankle bones

With your left fingers resting on the outside and your right fingers on the inside of the right ankle bone, firmly yet sensitively circle around each bone simultaneously (Figure 3.4). Repeat on the left foot to loosen any rigidity in the recipient's approach to life.

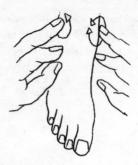

Figure 3.4 *Circle the ankle bones.*

Step 6 – shake the foot

Rest the mounds at the bases of both thumbs, in the hollows either side of the recipient's right ankle, just beneath the ankle bones (Figure 3.5). To shake the foot, keep the mounds of your hands in the same position, while moving your one hand towards the recipient and the other, in the opposite direction; then reverse this action. Watch the foot move from side to side. Once the right foot has had a good shake, repeat on the left foot. Effectively loosening the ankles makes it so much easier to adapt to life's ups and downs, as well as be more flexible and forgiving within relationships.

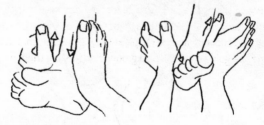

Figure 3.5 *Shake the feet.*

Step 7 – knead downwards

Gently rest the balls of the right toes against your right hand; make a loose fist with your left hand and place your knuckles just beneath the right toe necks. Knead firmly, but soothingly, all the way down, from the outer edge of the right foot to the tips of the heels (Figure 3.6) in a long, steady strip. Repeat strip by strip across the foot to the inner edge of the same foot. Reverse the role of your hands and repeat on the left foot to encourage the recipient to 'knuckle down' and get on with making the most of their life.

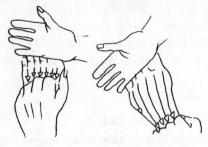

Figure 3.6 *Knead downwards.*

Step 8 – explore and release

Place all your fingertips, side by side, on top of the right toes (Figure 3.7) and make tiny circular movements over the top of the right foot, all the way up to the ankle crease; separate your hands so that the fingers continue massaging either side of the right ankle, to the back of the heels. Repeat the whole procedure three times, reducing your pressure each time, before moving over to their left foot and doing the same. This is a great way of easing any back tension and encouraging the recipient to let go of any unpleasantness that may be going on in the background and holding them back.

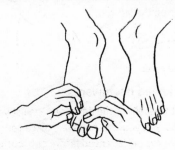

Figure 3.7 *Explore and release.*

Step 9 – pull the Achilles tendon

With the recipient lying as flat as possible, place your left hand under their right heel and your right hand on top of the same foot, in alignment with the foot and firmly 'pull' the right heel towards you (Figure 3.8) until a slight resistance is felt. Hold the stretch then very slowly release. Do this three times before repeating on their left foot to give the legs a good stretch and elongate the spine, releasing any unwanted tension or trapped nerves.

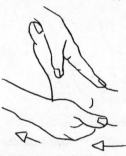

Figure 3.8 *Pull the Achilles tendon.*

Step 10 – stretch the foot

Take the recipient's right heel into your left hand, realign your right hand on top then gently, but firmly, bend their right foot downwards (Figure 3.9), stretching the upper surface as far as possible without resistance. Hold this stretch then allow the foot to slowly return to its natural position. Repeat three times and then do the same on the left foot.

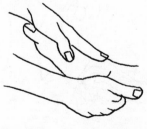

Figure 3.9 *Stretch the foot.*

Step 11 – rub the spinal reflexes

Use the heel of your right hand to caress the bony arch (Figure 3.10), first on the right foot, moving from the big toe to the ankle bone. Apply slight pressure as your hand eases its way up to the ankle bone, then lightly and slowly drag your hand back to their big toe. Repeat this a few times, before doing the same on their left arch, using the heel of your left hand to calm the nerves, get rid of inappropriate beliefs and encourage complete relaxation.

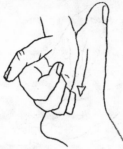

Figure 3.10 *Rub the spinal reflexes.*

In-between sequence

In between each sequence, cup both hands over the toes on the right foot, with your fingers on the top and thumbs underneath; then, with a loving squeeze, move your hands, simultaneously towards the ankles (Figure 3.11). Repeat three times on each foot to create overall harmony, accelerate healing and reassure the recipient.

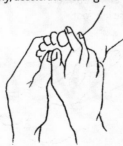

Figure 3.11 *In-between sequence.*

4

soothe the nerves and harmonize the endocrine system

Despite extreme negativity, fear and anxiety 'getting on the nerves', the brain is constantly tempted to entertain a host of self-limiting beliefs, intimidating self-talk and terrifying memories. Although this can be exceptionally detrimental and even debilitating, any negativity passing through the mind is transient. Meanwhile the endocrine system relies on the nervous system for information regarding any emotional shift so that together the two can detect and monitor what's going on. They differ though in that hormones act slowly but last longer, while nervous impulses respond quickly with almost instantaneous results. Massaging the endocrine system involves three important areas: the endocrine gland reflexes that need balancing, the circulatory reflexes for an uninterrupted blood flow and the target cell to ensure that the hormones are picked up and utilized beneficially. In this way, inner harmony and peace can be established and maintained throughout.

The nervous system

Always massage the nervous system reflexes immediately after the warm-up because the brain controls the functioning of the whole body. With the mind calm, the recipient is relieved of any fear or anxiety and their body can relax.

Step 12 – open the energy flows

Gently place all your fingertips onto the tips of each of the corresponding toes, except for the big toes (Figure 4.1). Apply gentle pressure, hold for a few seconds, and then gradually ease the pressure until your fingertips are just resting above the toe surfaces.

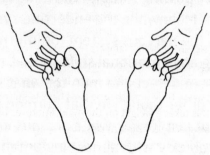

Figure 4.1 *Open the energy flows 1.*

Remove your fingers and lightly place the tips of your thumbs onto the tips of each big toe (Figure 4.2). Again apply slight

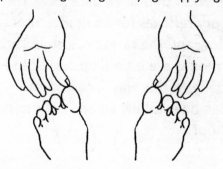

Figure 4.2 *Open the energy flows 2.*

pressure for a few seconds before gradually easing off, until your thumbs rest lightly or hover marginally above the big toes. The body may jerk and twitch as energy runs through it and you may also feel a delightful tingling or intense heat between your fingers and the recipient's toes; a sign that healing is actively taking place.

Step 13 – ease the mind

Simultaneously, rest your little fingers on the tips of the outer edges of the little toes (Figure 4.3). Gently push down for a few seconds, then ease off, lightly rotating your digits (Chapter 2) at the same time. Move your fingers fractionally along the tips of the little toes and repeat this pumping and rotating movement. Continue until the tops of both little toes have been well stimulated. Return your little fingers to the outer edges of the little toes but slightly lower down and continue the technique across all toe pads, from the little to the big toes, starting a fraction lower down every time until the toe pads have been thoroughly massaged. This takes a weight off the mind, improves brain activity, expands the capacity to think, makes more space for exciting new concepts, prolongs concentration and favourably alters thought patterns. By calming or exciting the hypothalamus, at the base

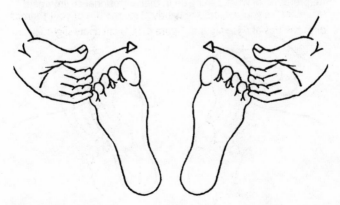

Figure 4.3 *Ease the mind.*

of the brain, it also affects the production and functioning of the hormones, for even greater inner harmony. It also rejuvenates the face.

Step 14 – improve the eyesight

Place your thumbs over the centres of both little toe pads, with your little fingers directly opposite, on top (Figure 4.4). Lightly squeeze the two digits together until a slight resistance is felt; hold for a few seconds then gently and slowly rotate your thumbs, while visualizing red. Gradually ease the pressure until there is little or no contact. Now lightly rest your little fingers on the hubs of the toe pads, over the eye reflexes, for a short while. Repeat the procedure on the mounds of the fourth toe pads, using your thumbs with your ring fingers, while visualizing orange; then on the mounds of the third toes, with your thumbs and middle fingers, with yellow in mind; then on the mounds of the second toes with your thumbs and index fingers, picturing green and, finally, on the hubs of the big toe pads, with your thumbs on the toe pads and your index fingers on top, imagining purple and blue. This technique is ideal for improving eyesight, sharpening vision, easing eye strain, broadening the outlook, clarifying perceptions, helping to focus better, maximizing optical functioning and balancing the recipient's interpretation of what's going on in their emotional environment.

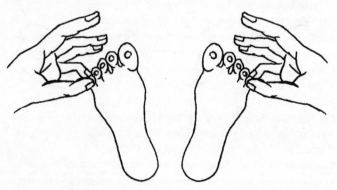

Figure 4.4 *Improve the eyesight.*

Step 15 – acknowledge the nose

Place your thumbs on the nose reflexes, on the inner joints of both big toes (Figure 4.5), with your middle fingers providing support on the opposite side. Gradually press the thumbs in, rotate them gently and then release. Now replace the thumbs with your middle fingers and rest them on these reflexes for a few seconds, visualizing yellow to enhance the sense of smell and encourage self-recognition. Acknowledging the nose keeps the recipient on track, doing what they should be doing and helps them to 'follow their nose'.

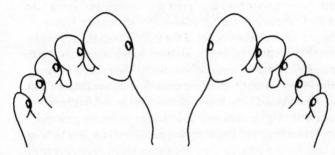

Figure 4.5 *Acknowledge the nose.*

Step 16 – for better hearing

Place your middle or little fingers on the outer joints of the recipient's little toes, over the ear reflexes (Figure 4.6), using your thumbs to support from the other side. Press and rotate (Chapter 2) for a few seconds, then gently squeeze the two digits together before lightly, but firmly, milking both sides simultaneously, from top to bottom, with a slight amount of compression between the two digits. Repeat on the fourth toes, using your ring fingers with your thumbs supporting; go on to the third toes, using your middle fingers and thumbs; move on to the second toes, with your index fingers and thumbs; and, finally, on to the big toes, but this time place your thumbs over the ear reflexes and use your middle fingers to support to enhance hearing, improve listening skills, create awareness of the inner mind chatter, make sounds clearer and clarify their meaning.

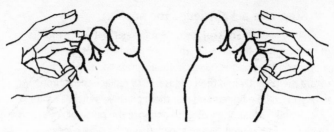

Figure 4.6 *For better hearing.*

Step 17 – soothe the mouth

Position your thumbs on the mouth reflexes (Figure 4.7), just beneath the inner joints of both big toes, placing your ring fingers on the opposite sides for support. Gradually press your thumbs in, then gently rotate before slowly releasing. Now place the tips of your ring fingers on both mouth reflexes for a few seconds, to facilitate speech, ease decision making, enhance self-confidence and for greater belief in personal concepts.

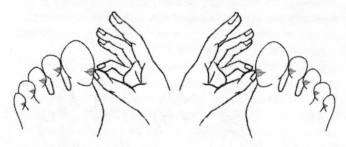

Figure 4.7 *Soothe the mouth.*

Step 18 – relax the jaw

Massage the jaw reflexes (Figure 4.8) using the rotation technique at the bases of each pair of toe pads to ease tension, prevent the grinding of teeth, increase mobility and the confidence to share innovative ideas with greater conviction.

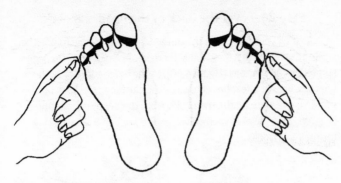

Figure 4.8 *Relax the jaw.*

Step 19 – milk the facial lymphatics

To milk the facial lymphatics, place your thumb pads side by side on the tip of the right little toe (Figure 4.9), then soothingly, yet firmly, stroke downwards, thumb over thumb, in tiny movements, from top to bottom. Do this several times until the right little toe pad is thoroughly milked. Now do the same on the fourth right toe, followed by the middle right toe, then the second right toe and eventually the big right toe. Repeat on the left toes to ease mental congestion and deeply ingrained impressions, opening the recipient's mind to every point of view.

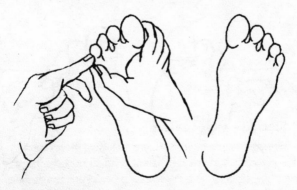

Figure 4.9 *Milk the facial lymphatics.*

Step 20 – over the back of the head and neck

Rest all your fingers on the outer edges of the little toes, either side of the recipient's feet. 'Walk' them in unison over the upper surfaces of all the toes (Figure 4.10), to the inner edges of both big toes. Repeat a few times to clear the clutter at the back of the mind, to evacuate fearful memories from the deep subconscious, to strengthen belief in themselves and to provide a firm backing for their own ideas.

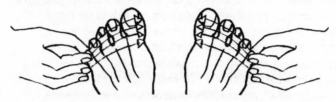

Figure 4.10 *Over the back of the head and neck.*

Open the avenues of expression

Step 21 – clear the throat

Place your thumbs onto the recipient's little toe necks, with your middle fingers on the other side (Figure 4.11). Gently squeeze the two digits together, hold for a while then gradually release

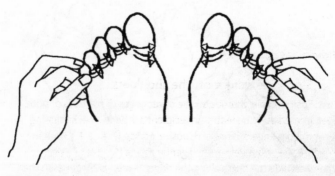

Figure 4.11 *Clear the throat.*

while, at the same time, lightly rotating (Chapter 2) with your thumbs, until there is little or no contact. Now do the same on the fourth toe necks with the thumbs and ring fingers; on the third toe necks with the thumbs and middle fingers; on the second toe necks with the thumbs and index fingers, finishing on the big toe necks.

Step 22 – caress the neck

Use your thumbs to gently, but firmly, stroke and milk the underneath surfaces of all toe necks, from top to bottom (Figure 4.12). Start on the right toe necks, going from the little to the big toe necks, then do the same on the left toe necks. Give additional attention to the sides, where there's often a lot of tension, due to unresolved emotions that remain unexpressed. Next feather stroke each toe neck, to continue easing neck and throat tension, assist lymph activity and increase blood flow to and from the head, opening up all the main avenues of self-expression.

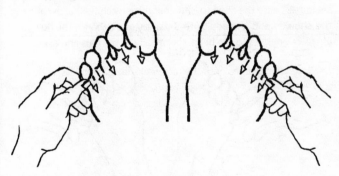

Figure 4.12 *Caress the neck.*

Step 23 – weight off the shoulders

Position your thumbs on the outer edges of the balls of both feet, immediately beneath the recipient's little toe necks, resting your middle fingers, directly opposite, on top (Figure 4.13). Lightly squeeze the two together then gently rotate (Chapter 2) your thumbs. Glide the digits along the ridge, immediately beneath the toe necks several times.

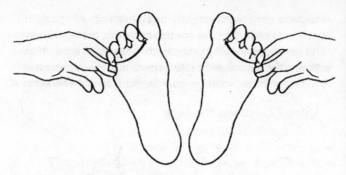

Figure 4.13 *A weight off the shoulders.*

Step 24 – ease the load

Gently but firmly slide your little fingers around the bases of each toe neck (Figure 4.14) before slipping them through the gaps going from the little to the big toes to take a 'weight off the shoulders', ease the need to 'shoulder responsibilities', allow all the 'shoulds' and 'shouldn'ts' to slip away and enhance the flow of life force energies to the head, specifically to the ears and eyes.

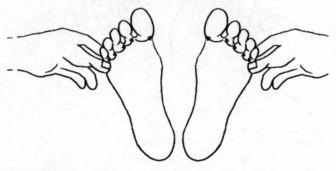

Figure 4.14 *Ease the load.*

Step 25 – release neck tension

Place all your fingers either side of the recipient's toe necks (Figure 4.15) and 'walk' them, in unison, over the tops of the toe necks to the inner edges of the big toe necks. Repeat two to three more times before milking. Now lightly run all your fingers (Figure 4.16), from the tips of the toes, over the tops of the feet, to the ankle creases to increase neck flexibility, to soothe the anxiety of 'getting it in the neck' or of feeling obliged to take on more than is really necessary or to clear anything hurtful or upsetting going on in the background.

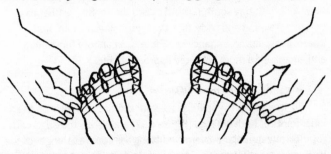

Figure 4.15 *Release neck tension.*

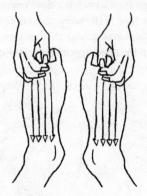

Figure 4.16 *Lightly run the fingers over the tops.*

Re-establish a firm backbone

The bony vertebrae of the spine are reflected along the hard 'knobbly' ridges of bone that extend from the inner joints of the big toes to just beneath the inner ankle bones. At the head of the spine is the midbrain, which synchronizes all the body's movements, breath and circulation.

Step 26 – co-ordinate mind and body

For the midbrain reflexes, place your thumbs or fingers on the tips of both big toes and gently massage down their inner edges to the joints, repeating a fraction to the top and then to the bottom of the strip so that the small area is thoroughly massaged. Now milk with tiny soothing strokes and then lightly feather to co-ordinate mind and body, fine-tune muscular co-ordination, improve respiration, enhance cardiac and circulatory functioning and encourage a more balanced approach to life.

Step 27 – ensure a firm backing

To strengthen the spine, place your thumbs or fingers on the inner joints of both big toes (Figure 4.17) and gently massage, with rotation or caterpillar movements, along the complete length of the bony ridges that border the insides of the feet. Finish just beneath the inner ankle bones; then repeat, but this time angle your thumbs downwards onto the tops of the bony ridges to stimulate or calm the sensory nerves. Repeat with your thumbs gently pushing upwards, underneath the bony ridges, so that the motor nerves are accessed. Milk the right spinal reflex, with small, repetitive soothing strokes, from the big toe to the ankle, and then the left spinal reflex.

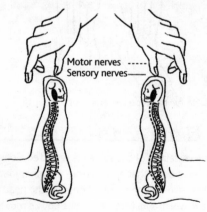

Figure 4.17 *Ensure a firm backing.*

Complete with an exceptionally light feathering, also from top to bottom, to either soothe agitated nerves or stimulate petrified nerves and facilitate the relay of nervous messages, while increasing each cell's awareness of its environment.

Step 28 – ease the neck

Repeat step 27, from the joints of the big toes to their bases (Figure 4.18), particularly for neck problems, so that flexibility is increased for every point of view to be clearly seen.

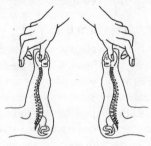

Figure 4.18 *Ease the neck.*

Step 29 – caress the upper back

Repeat step 27, but now go along the inner edges of both balls of the feet (Figure 4.19), to provide greater emotional strength.

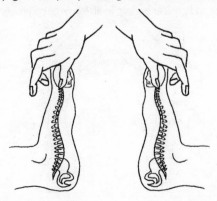

Figure 4.19 *Caress the upper back.*

Step 30 – strengthen the upper middle back

Repeat step 27, from the bases of the balls of the feet to both waistlines of the feet (Figure 4.20), for the strength to keep going, no matter what!

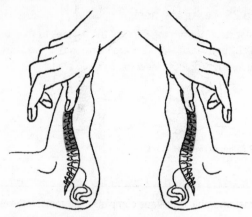

Figure 4.20 *Strengthen the upper middle back.*

Step 31 – reassure the lower middle back

Repeat step 27, from the waistlines of both feet to the junctions where the insteps and heels meet (Figure 4.21), for sound relationships and greater backup in all forms of communication.

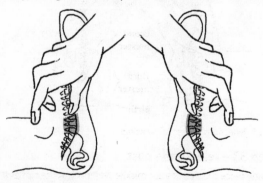

Figure 4.21 *Reassure the lower middle back.*

Step 32 – empower the lower back

Repeat step 27, around the bases of the inner ankles (Figure 4.22), to ease lower back pain and for greater inner resourcefulness.

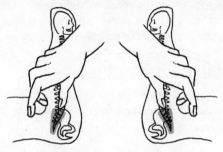

Figure 4.22 *Empower the lower back.*

The metamorphic technique

The metamorphic technique completes the spinal reflexes procedure by effectively liberating past fears and anxieties, particularly those experienced while in the womb (Figure 4.23).

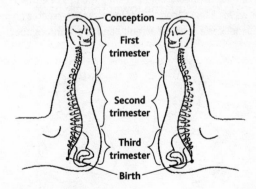

Figure 4.23 *Reflections of time in the womb.*

Step 33 – release the past

Lightly place the tips of your middle fingers onto the tips of the big toes; these points represent the time of conception. As you visualise a beautiful white light and take in three long deep breaths, glide your fingers slowly, barely touching the skin's surface, along the spinal reflexes, to just below the inner ankles, which symbolize the time of birth. Repeat another two to three times to effectively cut the invisible umbilical cord between the recipient and their mother, freeing them both of the need to be caught up in each other's energy.

The solar plexus technique

The solar plexus reflexes are the most powerful on the feet and can be massaged at any time to calm the recipient, should they panic for any reason.

Step 34 – create a centre of calm

Place both thumbs on the hollows (Figure 4.24) immediately beneath the balls of the feet and apply a gentle, but firm, pressure until a slight resistance is felt. Keep your thumbs still for a while and then gradually ease off, until the tips of your thumbs barely touch the skin's surface. Lightly stroke the reflexes either with your thumbs or middle fingers, before resting the tips of either digit on the hollows for a few seconds. This immediately creates an inner calm and induces a sense of serenity and peace throughout.

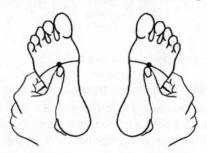

Figure 4.24 *Create a centre of calm.*

Complete the massage of the nervous system with the in-between sequence (Chapter 3) to create overall balance and harmony.

The endocrine system

The endocrine reflexes are generally quite sensitive, especially when there's a related issue.

Step 35 – put the pituitary gland back in control

Lightly drop your thumbs onto the upper ledges of the inner joints of both big toes (Figure 4.25). Apply gentle pressure, while gyrating your thumbs at the same time; then hold your thumbs still for a while before gradually easing off the pressure. Now place the tips of your middle fingers on these reflexes and lightly rest them here for a few seconds, while visualizing violet for greater clarity to calm the emotions, create inner harmony and balance the hormonal secretions, which improve the overall functioning of all the endocrine glands.

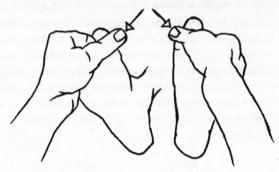

Figure 4.25 *Put the pituitary gland back in control.*

Step 36 – gain insight through the pineal gland

Rest your thumbs on the central mounds of both little toe pads (Figure 4.26) with your little fingers placed directly opposite. Squeeze the two digits gently together and then gradually release, while rotating with the thumbs. Now remove your thumbs. Lightly rest the tips of your index fingers in their place. Repeat on each toe mound, visualizing indigo to harmonize the natural cycle, regulate the menstrual cycle, stabilize mood swings, enhance intuition and enlighten mind, body and soul.

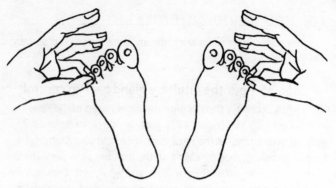

Figure 4.26 *Gain insight through the pineal gland.*

Step 37 – make space for the thyroid gland

Place your thumbs on the inner edges of the creases, at the bases of the big toes (Figure 4.27). Gently press down, hold for a while, and then, as you ease the pressure, lightly rotate. Replace your thumbs with the tips of your index fingers; resting them here for a short while and visualizing an exquisite turquoise blue. Now soothingly stroke the thyroid reflexes with your index fingers, to reduce the anxiety of trying to get on top of situations and for balance to be restored.

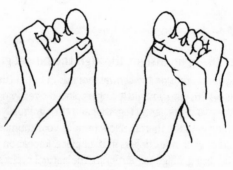

Figure 4.27 *Make space for the thyroid gland.*

Step 38 – reconnect with the spirit via the thymus gland

Feel for slight indentations or possible swellings, halfway down the inner edges of both balls of the recipient's feet. Rest your thumbs here, with your index fingers positioned directly opposite (Figure 4.28). Now gently squeeze the digits together and hold for a few seconds. As you ease the pressure, slowly rotate your thumbs; replace them with your index fingers while visualizing green; then lightly stroke with these fingers to encourage the recipient to really believe in themselves and boost their immunity.

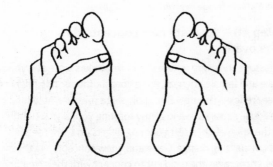

Figure 4.28 *Reconnect with the spirit via the thymus gland.*

Step 39 – finding courage through the adrenals

Place your thumbs or middle fingers on the adrenal gland reflexes (Figure 4.29), with your right digit slightly further in and fractionally lower down than your left. Apply minimal pressure and hold briefly before releasing, using the rotation technique. Gently milk with your thumbs; then feather caress with your middle fingers; now lightly rest the tips of these fingers on the adrenal gland reflexes for a few seconds, visualizing yellow to put the recipient at ease and give them the courage to implement their extraordinary and often unbelievable concepts, no matter what others say or think.

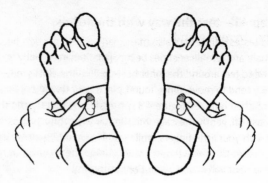

Figure 4.29 *Find courage through the adrenal glands.*

Step 40 – generate new concepts through the ovaries

Massage the ovary reflexes on both genders since everybody has male and female energies. Place your thumbs or ring fingers on the ovary reflexes (Figure 4.30), apply slight pressure, hold for a while, then gradually ease off while gently rotating your digits. Lightly stroke the reflexes, then rest your ring fingers on them for a few seconds, visualizing orange. Generating new concepts, via the ovarian reflexes, encourages the recipient to connect with their creative juices, as well as their gentler, more sensitive feminine qualities.

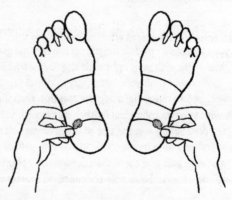

Figure 4.30 *Generate new concepts through the ovaries.*

Step 41 – test the way with the testes

The testes reflexes are also massaged on both genders because of the male and female energies being present in everybody. You may need to feel around the inner heels to find the testes reflexes, since they tend to move. Once found, place your thumbs or little fingers on their reflexes (Figure 4.31), press down slightly and then, as you ease off, gently massage. Milk lightly with your thumbs; then feather with your little fingers, while visualizing red. This ensures that the testes test the way and make a worthwhile contribution to the betterment and advancement of humankind.

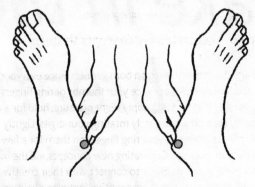

Figure 4.31 *Test the way with the testes.*

It's time, once again, for the 'in-between' sequence, detailed in Chapter 3, to enhance the overall effect of massaging the nervous and endocrine reflexes.

5

take in the breath of life

The respiratory system is influenced by innermost feelings about oneself and others, with excessive or unwanted emotions being constantly released through the breath. Disturbing notions, especially those related to the biological father, have a profound impact on the breathing process, along with fear, concern or anxiety, which cause the breath to be unconsciously suppressed or held. Overwhelming life circumstances that threaten personal well-being can even temporarily stop the breath. If the head and heart are in conflict, the resulting emotional havoc can lead to aggressive and sometimes destructive behaviour, with the reduced amount of oxygen having an adverse affect on the composition and functioning of the cells. Long term, this denies them of the opportunity to grow and develop naturally, with the lack of space and nourishment resulting in malformed cells. Reflexology encourages the recipient to take in deeper breaths of greater appreciation of themselves and other people.

The respiratory and cardiac system reflexes are massaged next to help the recipient to become reacquainted with their true spirit through the breath of life. Since these areas are linked to self-esteem and self-worth, massaging them also helps the recipient feel better about themselves and others.

Step 42 – expand the lungs

Place your thumbs immediately beneath the shoulder reflexes on the outer edges of the balls of both feet, with your index fingers directly opposite (Figure 5.1). Gently, but firmly, squeeze the two digits together and then slowly release, while lightly rotating your thumbs. Horizontally move both digits fractionally along and keep doing this, across the balls of the feet, to the bases of the big toes; now take your digits back to the outer edges, but, this time, place them a fraction lower down and massage the next horizontal strip. Continue doing this, strip by strip, all the way down until both balls of the feet have been thoroughly massaged. This expands the lung reflexes and ensures that there is plenty of space in which to breathe, allowing the recipient to adapt, more effortlessly, to the constant emotional changes within their environment.

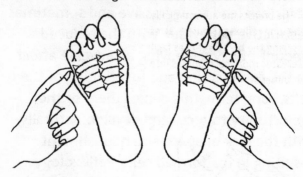

Figure 5.1 *Expand the lungs.*

Step 43 – take it all in

Rest your thumbs onto the balls of both feet, just below the little toes (Figure 5.2) and then either caterpillar or rotate downwards in vertical strips, from top to bottom, until both balls of the feet have been completely massaged. Now go to the outer edges of the right foot and milk firmly downwards, thumb over thumb, also in vertical strips, moving from the outside to the inside. Then, very lightly feather caress, in the same way, with your index fingers. Repeat on the ball of the left foot.

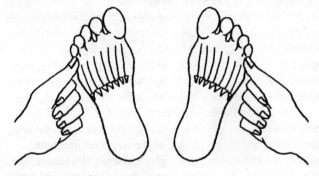

Figure 5.2 *Take it all in.*

Step 44 – keep abreast

The breasts are automatically caressed at the same time as the lung reflexes (Figure 5.3), easing any emotional congestion. Massaging the breast reflexes facilitates the nurturing process and creates more harmonious internal and external environments.

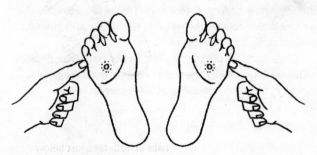

Figure 5.3 *Keep abreast.*

Step 45 – renew the love in the heart

Lightly place the tips of your index and middle fingers over the heart reflexes (Figure 5.4) on the inner edges, where the balls of the feet and insteps come together. Apply slight pressure for a while and then gradually ease off while gently rotating the digits. Rest for a moment before lovingly stroking these sensitive reflexes, while visualizing green or pink to enhance the effect.

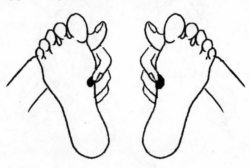

Figure 5.4 *Renew the love in the heart.*

Step 46 – firm up the ribcage

To massage the ribcage reflexes, place all your fingers either side of the balls of both feet. 'Walk' them several times, in unison, across the tops of both feet (Figure 5.5) from the outer to the inner edges; then, using the heels of your hands, gently caress the upper surfaces, this time going up the feet from the toes to the ankles. Finish by lightly running all your fingers in the same direction. The idea is to encourage the recipient to find the inner strength to emotionally back themselves.

Once again, it's time for the 'in-between' sequence, detailed in Chapter 2, to enhance the overall effect of massaging the respiratory and cardiac systems, as well as breast reflexes.

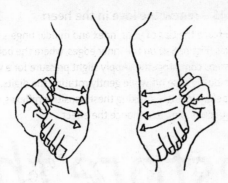

Figure 5.5 *Firm up the ribcage.*

6

restore the digestive system

Digestion is the way in which life's experiences are taken in, analysed, dealt with and absorbed so that the resultant energy can be used for further activities. Any unwanted, rough or wasteful aspects are fortunately eliminated. In this way, ongoing personal growth and development can be assured. However, it just takes a sudden change of mind or a fluctuation of an intense emotion, from extreme ecstasy to anger, fear, excitement, nervousness, insecurity, worry, apprehension or resistance, regarding what has happened or not happened, to immediately disturb the process. This is made worse when there's a build-up of resentment about having to take in or take on 'unpalatable' life experiences, or from having to digest extremely disagreeable and 'distasteful' situations. Massaging the digestive system reflexes eases the ultimate dissatisfaction and disappointment and restores everything to their natural state. In the process, the mind, body and spirit are re-energized and rejuvenated.

There are two parts to the digestive system; the accessory organs, which include the liver, pancreas and spleen, which aid digestion, based on past events, and the digestive tract itself, which processes things as they happen in the here and now.

Step 47 – enliven the liver

Place your left thumb on the outer edge of the right sole instep, immediately beneath the ball of the right foot, and your right thumb, a fraction lower down, on the opposite edge of the same foot (Figure 6.1). Either caterpillar or rotate your left thumb, horizontally across the sole instep, from the recipient's right to their left, to your right thumb. Place your left thumb back at the starting point but, this time, a little lower down, then keep it still as you massage towards it with your right thumb, from the inner to the outer edges of the right sole instep. Continue alternating the digits and massaging in both directions until the whole triangular reflex of the liver is thoroughly massaged. Now milk firmly downwards, thumb over thumb. Finish by lightly caressing the whole reflex with your third and ring fingers, from top to bottom. A tiny portion of the liver is reflected onto the left foot but this is massaged at the same time as the left stomach reflex, so it requires no specific action. Massaging the liver reflexes sorts out past events and gives the recipient the impetus to implement their own ideas for personal growth and development.

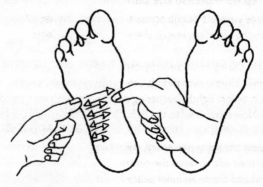

Figure 6.1 *Enliven the liver.*

Step 48 – have the gall

Rest your left thumb or third finger midway along the lower triangular edge of the liver reflex, on the right foot only (Figure 6.2). Gently rotate your digit on this minuscule ball-like reflex, then milk thumb over thumb in a downward movement, on the same spot. Lightly feather with your middle fingers to dissipate resentment and bitterness, making it possible to move on with peace of mind.

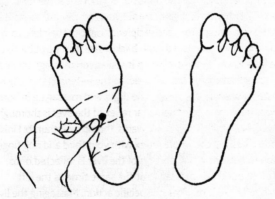

Figure 6.2 *Have the gall.*

Step 49 – please the pancreas

Place your left thumb across the left foot, immediately beneath the waistline; keep it there to use as a guideline (Figure 6.3). Now massage this tadpole-shaped reflex with your right thumb from the recipient's left to their right. Then firmly milk, thumb over thumb, across the reflex in the same direction, before lightly feathering downwards with your middle fingers. Now move over to the right foot, again placing your left thumb across the right foot immediately beneath the waistline and repeat the same procedure, still moving from the recipient's right to their left, as far as the centre of the foot to balance the pancreas and create an inner peace about all that is taking place.

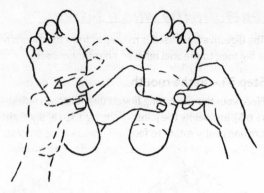

Figure 6.3 *Please the pancreas.*

Step 50 – surprise the spleen

With your thumbs either side of the spleen reflex (Figure 6.4), on the upper, outer quadrant of the recipient's left fleshy instep, gently caterpillar or rotate in both directions until the whole reflex has been thoroughly massaged. Then firmly milk downwards, thumb over thumb, before lightly feathering with your middle fingers for a more balanced approach to life.

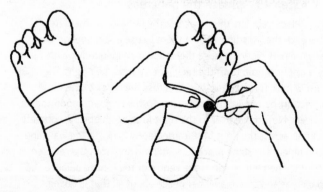

Figure 6.4 *Surprise the spleen.*

Re-energize the whole system

The digestive tract itself is massaged from the mouth reflexes, on the big toes, to the anal reflexes, on the inner heels.

Step 51 – in the mouth

Place your thumbs or ring fingers on the mouth reflexes (Figure 6.5), just below the joints of the big toes; apply slight pressure and gently rotate to facilitate the chewing process, improve the sense of taste and assist with decision making.

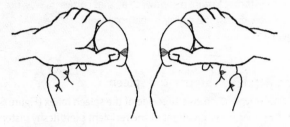

Figure 6.5 *In the mouth.*

Step 52 – soothe the oesophagus

Caterpillar with your thumbs or index fingers from the mouth reflexes all the way down the inner edges of the balls of both feet (Figure 6.6) several times before lightly milking with your thumbs.

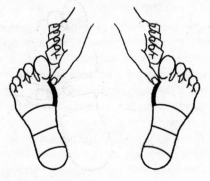

Figure 6.6 *Soothe the oesophagus.*

Finish by gently feather stroking with your index fingers, to pacify or excite the peristaltic action to ease the taking in and swallowing of life's experiences with greater understanding.

Step 53 – open the stomach

Massage the cardiac sphincter reflexes (Figure 6.7), at the entrance of the stomach, by resting your thumbs or index fingers on both reflexes and applying slight pressure; hold for a few seconds, then gradually release. Now gently stroke thumb over thumb to make the stomach more receptive to all that comes its way, no matter how distasteful it may sometimes seem.

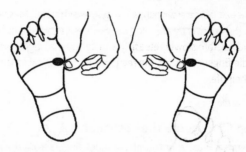

Figure 6.7 *Open the stomach.*

Step 54 – rub the tummy

Visualize the stomach reflex in the upper, inner quadrant of the left foot (Figure 6.8) then, using either the caterpillar or rotation technique, massage it horizontally, either with your thumbs or middle fingers, going from one side of the reflex to the other to mimic the churning movement of the stomach. Next milk horizontally, thumb over thumb, towards the right foot, before feathering in the same direction, with your middle fingers. Now massage the small portion of stomach reflex on the right foot, this time going from the recipient's left to their right to assist in 'stomaching' and coping with life's ongoing experiences.

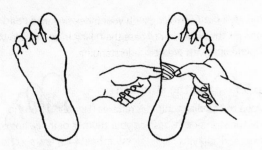

Figure 6.8 *Rub the tummy.*

Step 55 – move it on

At the exit of the stomach is the pyloric sphincter. Massage this reflex (Figure 6.9) by applying slight pressure, then hold for a few seconds, before slowly releasing and lightly massaging with your middle fingers to assist the recipient in moving on to the next stage of their life.

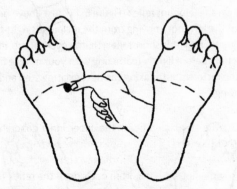

Figure 6.9 *Move it on.*

Step 56 – around the 'C' of the duodenum

Use your right thumb to massage the C-shaped duodenum reflex, only on the inner, upper quadrant of the right foot (Figure 6.10) changing your thumbs midway to make the movement flow better.

Then lightly milk the 'C' before gently feathering with your middle fingers to assist the recipient in dealing with past issues so that they can get on and enjoy the present.

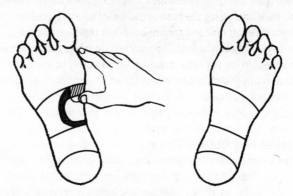

Figure 6.10 *Around the 'C' of the duodenum.*

Step 57 – cajole the jejunum

Massage the jejunum reflex (Figure 6.11), just above or on the waistline of the left foot, moving from the recipient's right to their left. Now gently milk this short reflex, thumb over thumb, in the same direction, before lightly feathering with your middle fingers to cajole the recipient into taking the next exciting step and keep things moving.

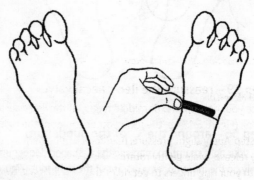

Figure 6.11 *Cajole the jejunum.*

Step 58 – wind through the small intestines

Place your right thumb at the start of the small intestine reflex (Figure 6.12), then massage horizontally from the recipient's left to their right, using the base of the waistline as a guideline. Go from their left foot and continue on their right foot. At the outer edge of their right foot, use your left thumb to return across both insteps in the opposite direction, immediately beneath the previous horizontal strip. Continue, backwards and forwards, from one side to the other, until both lower sole insteps have been thoroughly massaged. Now lightly milk with your thumbs, in the same way, then gently feather stroke the whole area with your ring fingers for greater tolerance and understanding within relationships.

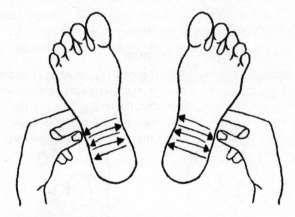

Figure 6.12 *Wind through the small intestines.*

Step 59 – reassure the ileo-caecal valve

Place your right thumb or middle finger on the ileo-caecal valve reflex (Figure 6.13), in the lower, outer corner of the right fleshy instep. Apply slight pressure, hold for a while, then gradually release, while gently rotating. Now lightly stroke the reflex with your ring fingers to get rid of the old and make way for the new.

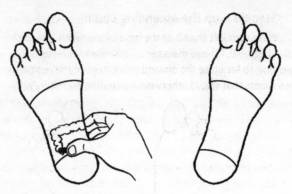

Figure 6.13 *Reassure the ileo-caecal valve.*

Step 60 – clear out the appendix

Place your left thumb or fourth finger on the appendix reflex (Figure 6.14), found only on the recipient's right foot. Massage this minuscule reflex with tiny rotational movements, then lightly stroke with your ring fingers to help those who feel that their life is going nowhere, along with those caught up in a dead-end relationship or job.

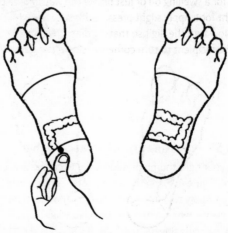

Figure 6.14 *Clear out the appendix.*

Step 61 – up the ascending colon

Place your left thumb at the base of the ascending colon reflex (Figure 6.15) and massage up the reflex, as far as the waistline, to facilitate the onward movement of the remnants of life's events that would otherwise waste time and energy.

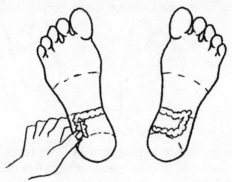

Figure 6.15 *Up the ascending colon.*

Step 62 – around the hepatic flexure

Feel for a swelling on or just below the waistline (Figure 6.16) of the right foot. Apply slight pressure, hold it for a while and then release. Now turn the digit so that it points towards the left foot. It helps the recipient to turn corners with greater ease.

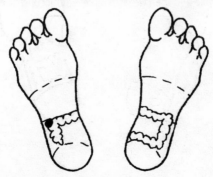

Figure 6.16 *Around the hepatic flexure.*

Step 63 – across the transverse colon

Massage the transverse colon reflexes (Figure 6.17), following the base of the waistline, from the hepatic flexure reflex on the right foot to the centre of the left foot, going slightly upwards, towards the splenic flexure on the outer edge of the left sole instep to relieve the pressure of having to perform and meet unreasonably high expectations.

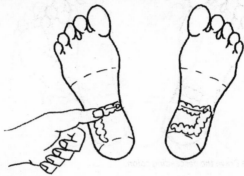

Figure 6.17 *Across the transverse colon.*

Step 64 – around the splenic flexure

With your left thumb, feel for the slight swelling of the splenic flexure reflex (Figure 6.18) and massage it well. Now turn your right thumb so that it's angled downwards and apply slight pressure. Hold for a while and then release to prevent hiccups.

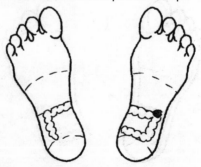

Figure 6.18 *Around the splenic flexure.*

Step 65 – down the descending colon

With your right thumb, still pointing downwards, massage down the outer border of the left instep to the heel (Figure 6.19), to get wasteful remnants moving along the descending colon.

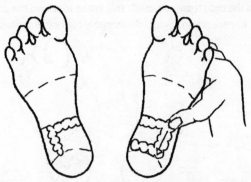

Figure 6.19 *Down the descending colon.*

Step 66 – skirt the sigmoid flexure

Rest your right thumb on the sigmoid flexure reflex, in the lower corner of the left sole instep (Figure 6.20), and apply slight pressure. Hold this for a while and then release. Now turn your thumb so that it's pointing towards the inside edge of the left foot.

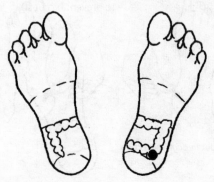

Figure 6.20 *Skirt the sigmoid flexure.*

Step 67 – slither along the sigmoid colon

Slither your right thumb along the sigmoid colon reflex, at the base of the left sole instep, just above the heel pad, going from the recipient's left to their right (Figure 6.21) to keep remnants moving and help them on their way out.

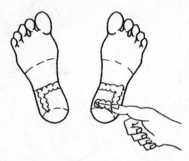

Figure 6.21 *Slither along the sigmoid colon.*

Step 68 – out through the rectum

Massage the arcs of the rectum reflexes by placing your thumbs or little fingers on the inner edges of both feet, at the junction where the heels and insteps meet (Figure 6.22), to ease the release of all the rough aspects of life.

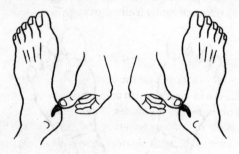

Figure 6.22 *Out through the rectum.*

Step 69 – angling for the anus

Apply slight pressure to the anus reflexes (Figure 6.23), hold it for a few seconds, and now release for the utter relief of totally letting go and, in so doing, complete the digestive process.

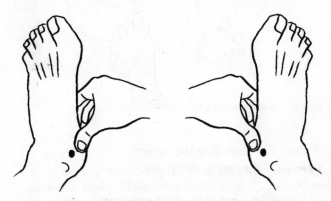

Figure 6.23 *Angling for the anus.*

Step 70

Firmly milk, thumb over thumb, the complete length of the large colon, from the ascending colon (Step 61) to the anus (Step 69), then lightly feather stroke with the fourth fingers.

Step 71 – over the middle back

Place all your fingers on the outer edges of both insteps (Figure 6.24) and 'walk' them in unison over the tops, from the outsides of the feet to the insides. Repeat several times, then lightly run the tips of your fingers up the feet, from the bases of all the toes to the ankle creases to provide the inner strength to carry on.

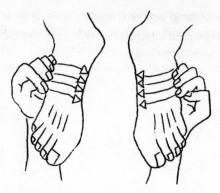

Figure 6.24 *Over the middle back.*

Step 72 – soothing the innards

Massage along the fleshy insteps on the inner edges of the feet (Figure 6.25), immediately below the bony arch. Now milk, with the heels of your hands, moving towards the recipient; finally, run all your fingers along these reflexes to ensure ongoing resourcefulness.

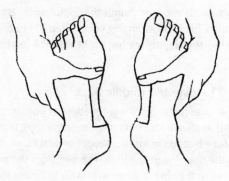

Figure 6.25 *Soothing the innards.*

It's time for the in-between sequence again, detailed in Chapter 2, to enhance the overall effect of the digestive procedure.

7

reinstate the bones, muscles and skin

There's a fascinating correlation between the skeletal, muscular, excretory and reproductive systems; all are influenced by inner security and social standing. The support received, along with the ability to get ahead are either enhanced or hindered by family and social beliefs. So it's necessary to have the strength to 'be one of a kind', to build up the bones, as well as be flexible enough in the mind to keep the muscles moving and get on and do things, regardless of what others say or think. En route there's bound to be things that waste time, sap resources or drain the whole of its energy, so the excretory system efficiently gets rid of anything that gets in the way, making room for exciting new concepts that can grow and develop, courtesy of the reproductive systems, to make a much-needed world of difference. Reflexology is one way to ensure that this happens.

Step 73 – strengthen the pelvis

Place your thumbs or little fingers onto the outer edges of both heel pads, where they join the insteps (Figure 7.1) and firmly caterpillar or rotate in horizontal strips, from the outer to the inner edges of both heels. Keep repeating this, moving your digits fractionally down each time, until both heels have been thoroughly massaged. Next milk downwards, thumb over thumb, from the outer to the inner edges, then lightly feather stroke with your little fingers for a more solid foundation, as well as greater mobility and flexibility, especially during childbirth.

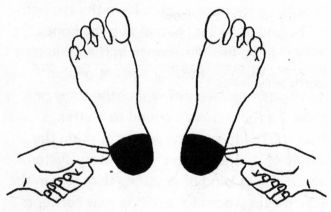

Figure 7.1 *Strengthen the pelvis.*

Restrengthen the limbs

Step 74 – along the upper arm reflexes

Place your thumbs or index fingers immediately below the little toes and simultaneously massage along the outer edges of the balls of both feet (Figure 7.2) to the elbow reflexes. Now firmly milk, thumb over thumb, and then feather caress with your little fingers for greater confidence in reaching out and embracing new beginnings.

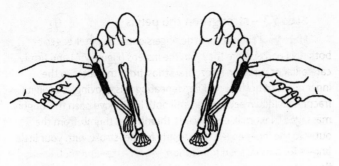

Figure 7.2 *Along the upper arm reflexes.*

Step 75 – flex the elbows

Generously massage the elbow reflexes (Figure 7.3), the prominent bones midway down the outer edges of both feet; then firmly milk them, before lightly feathering, to give the recipient room to be themselves.

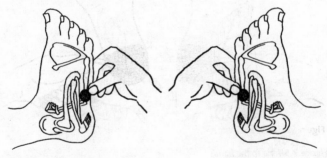

Figure 7.3 *Flex the elbows.*

Step 76 – down the lower arm

Use your thumbs to massage the lower arm reflexes (Figure 7.4), along the outside edges of both feet at a 45° angle, between the elbow and hand reflexes. Now firmly milk along these reflexes, thumb over thumb, then caress lightly with your middle fingers to assist with coping with anything that has been kept 'at arm's length'.

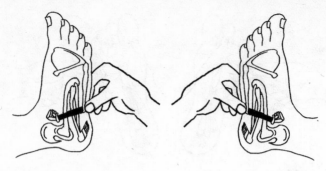

Figure 7.4 *Down the lower arm.*

Step 77 – tend to the hands

Tend to the hands (Figure 7.5) in the same way as the elbow reflexes (step 75), making it easier to handle life.

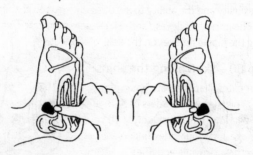

Figure 7.5 *Tend to the hands.*

Step 78 – up the thighs

Rest your thumbs on the knee reflexes (Figure 7.6) then caterpillar or rotate your digits up towards the base of the outer ankle bones. Now milk with both thumbs, then stroke lightly with your ring finger to be more open to life's opportunities and move on when necessary.

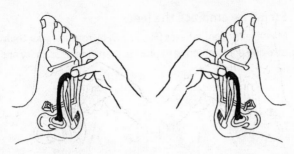

Figure 7.6 *Up the thighs.*

Step 79 – knead the knees

Feel for the tiny bony ledges, just above the midway point between the shoulder and elbow reflexes; these are secondary accesses to the knees. Apply slight pressure, release and massage thoroughly, then stroke lightly with your middle fingers to encourage greater flexibility and the ability to adapt to unexpected changes of direction. The primary reflexes, for the knees, are stimulated when massaging the nipple reflexes on the balls of the feet.

Step 80 – skim along the shins

Either caterpillar or rotate your thumbs along the shin reflexes (Figure 7.7) on the outer borders of both feet, from the knee to the feet reflexes. Now milk thoroughly with your thumbs, then gently feather stroke with your index fingers for the strength to follow through with worthwhile activities.

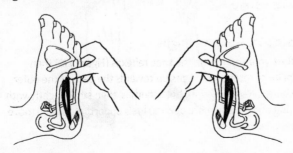

Figure 7.7 *Skim along the shins.*

Step 81 – embrace the feet

Massage the foot reflexes (Figure 7.8) by rotating your thumbs, then stroking and feathering to provide even greater stability and mobility.

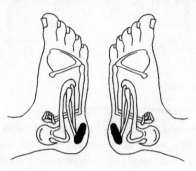

Figure 7.8 *Embrace the feet.*

Step 82 – bolster the buttocks

Caress the buttock reflexes (Figure 7.9) several times on the outer triangular areas of both heels either with your thumbs or all your fingers. Then soothe these areas with the heels of your hands, before lightly feathering with all your fingers. Bolstering the buttock reflexes helps strengthen the seat of power.

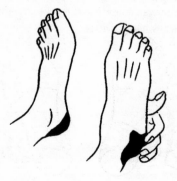

Figure 7.9 *Bolster the buttocks.*

Step 83 – reinforce the hips

Circle around the hip reflexes (Figure 7.10), on the outer ankle bones, with either your thumbs or all your fingers, first firmly, then lightly, to provide the impetus and force needed to move ahead with ease.

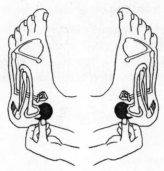

Figure 7.10 *Reinforce the hips.*

Appease the reproductive organs

Step 84 – attend to the fallopian tubes

Place your thumbs or ring fingers on the ovary reflexes (Figure 7.11) and massage from the outer to the inner aspects of

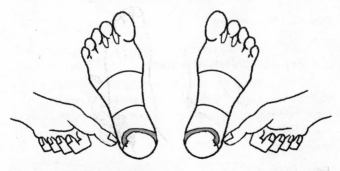

Figure 7.11 *Attend to the fallopian tubes.*

the lower fleshy insteps, with gentle rotation movements. Next lightly milk thumb over thumb, then gently feather stroke with your ring fingers, to clear the way for new ideas to come through.

Step 85 – from the other side

Now massage the secondary fallopian tube reflexes from the other side (Figure 7.12) this time by caterpillaring, then milking, from the outer to the inner ankle bones, along the ankle creases, to further assist in bringing new concepts out into the open.

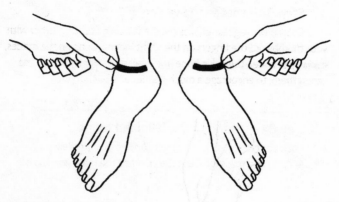

Figure 7.12 *From the other side.*

Step 86 – unleash the uterus

Gently massage the uterus reflexes (Figure 7.13) with your thumbs or little fingers, then lightly stroke and caress them, especially during pregnancy, to create a more harmonious environment within the home, as well as balance the feminine energy.

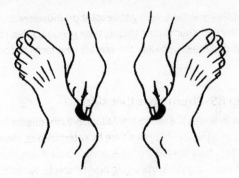

Figure 7.13 *Unleash the uterus.*

Step 87 – soothe the vagina

Soothe the vaginal reflexes (Figure 7.14), by rotating either with your thumbs or little fingers on the slight indentations on the insides, midway between the ankle bone and heels; then lightly stroke and caress them, to encourage a much gentler approach to life.

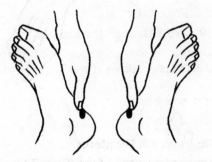

Figure 7.14 *Soothe the vagina.*

Step 88 – bolster manly assets

Thoroughly massage the inner triangular areas on both heels (Figure 8.15), either with your thumbs or with all of your fingers; now milk well, then feather with your little fingers for greater inner strength, enhanced personal performance and to make the recipient feel important, so that they can rise appropriately to any occasion.

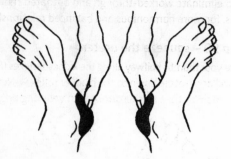

Figure 7.15 *Bolster manly assets.*

It's time once again for the 'in-between' sequence, detailed in Chapter 2, to enhance the effect of reflexology on the limb, buttock and lower reproductive organs and glands.

Release the past

Step 89 – work through the kidneys

Place your thumbs, or ring fingers, pointing downwards, at the top of both kidney reflexes (Figure 7.16) and massage

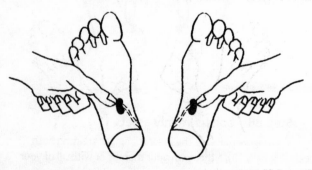

Figure 7.16 *Work through the kidneys.*

the tiny strips of about an inch, from top to bottom, either by caterpillaring or rotating your digits. Next milk thoroughly with your thumbs, then feather stroke with your middle and ring fingers to eliminate worked-through and outdated thoughts and emotions, for more harmonious and balanced relationships.

Step 90 – squeeze the ureters

Place your thumbs halfway along the kidney reflexes (Figure 7.17) and caterpillar or rotate down to the bladder reflexes. Now milk with your thumbs, then feather stroke with your ring fingers.

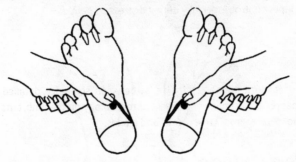

Figure 7.17 *Squeeze the ureters.*

Step 91 – reassure the bladder

Rest your thumbs or little fingers on the fleshy mounds at the bases of the inner heels (Figure 7.18) and gently palpate these reflexes.

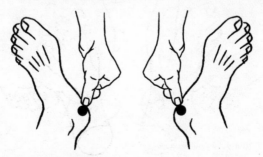

Figure 7.18 *Reassure the bladder.*

Now lightly milk them, and then tenderly feather stroke them with your little fingers to help the bladder be more accommodating.

Step 92 – aid the flow

Place your thumbs or little fingers at the start of the urethra reflexes on the edges of the fleshy mounds (Figures 7.19 and 7.20) and massage to the tips of the inside heels on men and to the midway hollow on women. Concentrate on the slight indentations on females and on the tips of the heels on males. Now firmly milk with your thumbs, then gently feather stroke with your little fingers for inner control, especially during distressing periods.

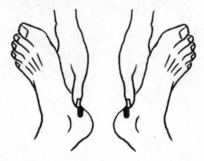

Figure 7.19 *Aid the flow on females.*

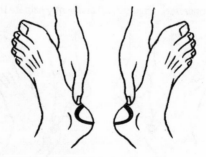

Figure 7.20 *Aid the flow on males.*

Now do the in-between sequence, detailed in Chapter 2, to enhance the overall effect of massaging the excretory system.

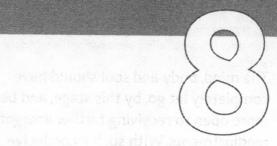

8
the finale

The mind, body and soul should have completely let go, by this stage, and be more open to receiving further energetic readjustments. With such a conducive environment for healing, the finale ensures that the state of homoeostasis continues and is preserved for as long as possible. This is a valuable opportunity to be rid of all the usual problems and be lifted from self-limiting circumstances. With reflexology being the key to relaxation, it opens the mind to greater concepts, calms the whole body and soothes ruffled emotions. By utilizing the natural energy flows, the body is able to make the most of its own marvellous recuperative abilities to get better. Reflexology is perfect for putting life back into perspective and pointing the feet in the best direction for self-empowerment and self-actualization. The resultant feeling of well-being and overall harmony can then radiate outwardly to positively affect others and ultimately the world.

By this time, the recipient should be completely relaxed, making it an ideal opportunity to gently stretch and extend the feet for greater flexibility and expansion of mind, body and soul.

Step 93 – stretch the mind and spine

Gently pull both little toes simultaneously (Figure 8.1) then release; now pull the fourth toes and let go; do the same on the third toes, the second toes and finally the big toes. Gently tug the big toes for slightly longer to relieve neck tension, headaches, back disorders and open the recipient to the many possibilities available to them.

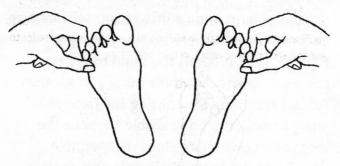

Figure 8.1 *Stretch the mind and spine.*

Step 94 – extend the neck

Lightly support the base of the right little toe, between your left thumb and index finger, then take the right little toe between your right thumb and index finger and rotate it, first anti-clockwise and then clockwise (Figure 8.2). Do the same with the fourth right toe, and then with each toe, one by one. Now repeat on the left foot, starting with the left little toe and finishing with the left big toe. Spend extra time on rotating both big toes since it effectively eases neck tension and loosens up mind and body.

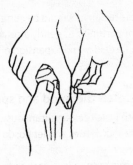

Figure 8.2 *Extend the neck.*

Step 95 – flex the upper body

Place your hands either side of the recipient's right foot and gently roll it from side to side (Figure 8.3); repeat on the left foot to facilitate the give and take in life and, in so doing, make it easier to expand and contract, which, in turn, boosts the morale.

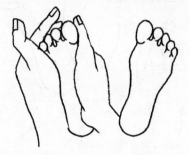

Figure 8.3 *Flex the upper body.*

Step 96 – extend the whole being

With both hands on top of the recipient's feet, gently, but firmly, stretch the feet downwards, hold for a while (Figure 8.4) and then release. Next place the palms of your hands flat against both soles and coax the feet upwards. This simple technique is great for broadening horizons and encourages a more amenable approach to life.

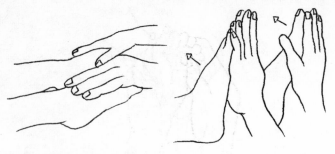

Figure 8.4 *Extend the whole being.*

Step 97 – relax the lower torso

Support the right heel with your left hand and use your right hand to rotate the right foot, as fully as possible, first anti-clockwise and then clockwise (Figure 8.5). Change hands and repeat on the left foot. This relaxes the lower torso, balancing the odds and keeping life events in proportion.

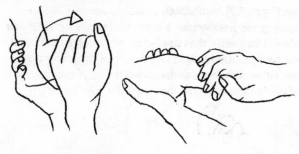

Figure 8.5 *Relax the lower torso.*

Step 98 – loosen up

Place your thumbs together, immediately beneath the right middle toe neck, with your fingers resting on top (Figure 8.6); then gently push up with your thumbs, while using your fingers to lightly stretch the top of the foot over the soles. Repeat this several times, as your hands gradually progress all the way down the middle portion of the right foot. Now do the same on the left foot, to encourage

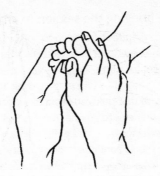

Figure 8.6 *Loosen up.*

a more relaxed and contented approach to life, while, at the same time, energizing the whole being.

Step 99 – the final step

Complete the reflexology sequence by massaging the solar plexus reflexes for a minute or two. Place your thumbs on the hollows (Figure 8.7), immediately beneath the balls of the feet, and apply gentle pressure until a slight resistance is felt. Keep your thumbs still for a while, then slowly ease off, until the tips of your thumbs barely touch the skin's surface. Now lightly stroke the reflexes, either with your thumbs or middle fingers, then rest the tips of your middle fingers on the hollows for a few seconds.

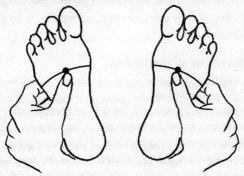

Figure 8.7 *The final step.*

Step 100 – bringing the session to an end

Stroke first the right foot, from top to bottom, and then the left foot in the same way. Cover both feet, and then continue to hold the covered feet for a little longer. As you do so, use a soft voice to invite the recipient to take in three deep breaths, before opening their eyes, so that they can begin to surface in their own time. A glass of water helps to ground them, as well as flush out their system and enhance the effect of having their feet massaged, which is why they should continue to drink plenty of water. Also suggest that they wrap up well, especially if it's cold outside, since a tremendous amount of heat can be lost, during and after a treatment, because of being so relaxed.

First-aid reflexology

Ideally always give a complete massage on both feet to ensure overall wellbeing through homeostasis of mind, body and soul. Occasionally, however, when there is insufficient time, giving a quick massage is better than nothing. This entails massaging all the toes thoroughly (steps 12–25), soothing the spinal reflexes (steps 26–32), pacifying the solar plexus reflexes (step 34) and balancing the energy centres (steps 35–41). Always finish with the 'in between' massage (Chapter 2) of both feet. Should there be a particular discomfort in the body, massage its related reflex or reflexes as well. End the short massage by soothing the solar plexus reflexes (step 34).

If you are at all concerned

If, at any time, you are at all concerned, or the recipient panics for any reason, then immediately place your thumbs on their solar plexus reflexes and ask them to take in long, deep breaths. Guide them into relaxing more and more with each out breath, reassuring them that the reaction is only temporary and it's a good sign that a favourable shift has taken place. If it's available, also give them a few drops of rescue remedy.